# Body Butters For Beginners:

## BY LINDSEY P

# Proven Secrets To Making All Natural Body Butters For Rejuvenating And Hydrating Your Skin

### 2nd Edition

# Table Of Contents

# Introduction

I want to thank you and congratulate you for purchasing the book, *"Body Butters For Beginners: Proven Secrets To Making All Natural Body Butters For Rejuvenating And Hydrating Your Skin"*
This book contains proven steps and strategies on how to have radiant and healthy skin with the help of body butters, which you can make all by yourself and at the comfort of your home.

Do you know that having healthy and beautiful skin is as easy as ABC? With simple to follow steps, you can make your own body butters! Whether you are a beginner or an expert chef, you can dish out a body butter recipe for you and your loved ones – not to be eaten of course, but to be applied on the skin. Say goodbye to dry, scaly skin and start giving your skin the star treatment it deserves.

Thanks again for purchasing this book, I hope you enjoy it!

# Chapter 1 Deeper Than Skin Deep

## Deeper Than Skin Deep

### *Healthy skin equals a healthy you*

Beautiful skin makes all the difference when it comes to total physical beauty. How could it not? The skin is the largest organ of the body and you simply can't avoid seeing it.

When you see famous celebrities in movies and on TV, the first thing you would usually notice about them is their flawless skin. These stars know the importance of taking care of their skin. It is not just superficial for them.

The care for the skin is from inside out. Well, you are a star in your own right and your skin deserves that star treatment as well. You would not regret all the time and finances you spend on taking care of your skin. It would glow and people would know. A healthy skin is something you cannot hide.

How does one achieve an overall great and healthy skin? First, get to know the skin very well. What is it? What is it made of? What does it need?

### *Your first line of defense*

Skin is very important in protecting you and everything inside your body. Imagine, if you do not have skin? It would be gross to see the muscles, bones, and organs all out, wouldn't it? And you would not last long what with all the foreign bodies and infections that might set in to your vital organs.

You could really say that the value of skin is really more than skin deep. It's technically life for everybody. Not only does it protect your body, it also helps your body maintain the right temperature. And without skin how would you be able to feel that tender touch of your loved ones?

Nobody can boast that he or she would survive without the help of the skin. So, maintaining it to be healthy is a must for all. This is, after all, your first line of defense against whatever is the enemy of the body.

What is skin made of? Let's find out.

### Parts of skin: three layers

1.  Epidermis – the outermost layer. This is what you can see and touch. If you look at the skin on your hand right now, it seems like nothing is going on in there, right? Do not be deceived. Just beneath it is a busy network of different cells and organisms with the sole purpose of making new skin cells. After 2 weeks or a month, these new skin cells would move up to the epidermis. As new cells arise, the old ones die and move on top of the epidermis where they would be shed off. Around 30k-40k of dead cells are being shed off every minute! Imagine, just by reading this alone, millions of cells have died and have been replaced already in your body. Could the body catch up on replacing these with new cells? You need not worry as the epidermis works 95% all the time to make new skin for you. The other 5% works for melanin. This gives the color of your skin. The darker you are, the more melanin is produced. This keeps you safe from the sun's harmful rays. They make extra melanin to protect you from being sunburned. However, your

skin cannot do it alone. It needs you to help protect itself from the destructive effects of the sun. You can do this by applying sunblock or using an umbrella or wearing a hat during a sunny day.

2. Dermis – lies just beneath the epidermis. This is where the blood vessels, nerves, sweat and oil glands are located. There is where you'll find the tough and stretchy collagen and elastin. Nerve endings help you to feel –whether what you have touched was hot or cold. The blood vessels deliver and supply nutrients and oxygen to the skin. Oil or sebaceous glands produce the skin's natural oil called sebum. This body's oil protects and lubricates the skin. Sebum acts as the body's waterproof shield. Have you seen water and oil mix? Sebum makes sure you won't absorb so much water that your skin would be soggy. Sweat glands protect the skin too. They came through pores or the tiny holes in the skin.

3. Subcutaneous fat –the bottom part of the skin, which is mostly made of fat. It helps the body to be warm. It also absorbs shock if you fall down or hit something. This is where the hair follicles are located, too.

### *Functions of the skin*

As you know by now, your skin protects the whole body. It also warms or cools you so that you maintain 37 degrees C or 98.6 degrees F which is the ideal temperature for the body. During a hot day, your body would release heat through the skin to cool you down. So you perspire a lot. When it is cold, your body would preserve heat to keep you warm.

The skin is really deeper than skin deep. It deserves special attention and care. There are many products that can help you moisturize and keep your skin healthy, supple and glowing. Learn more about them as you read on.

# Chapter 2 Which Is Which?

## Which is which?

Skin care and skin products flood the market. This is a growing industry, which is getting and getting more popular as the years pass. The consumers are sometimes confused which products would benefit them the most.

A lot of people are willing to spend so much just to have beautiful skin. They sometimes commit the error of just buying the most expensive product. Price is not necessarily the basis of how good a skin product is for your skin.

To get the most out of these skin products, you should first know your skin type. There are different skin types. The factors that may affect your skin type include the race, age, weather or season and your overall health status. If you cannot personally determine your skin type, then you can avail the help of the professionals. Your skin is worth it.

### *Assess your skin type.*

There are four skin types– dry, oily, normal and combination.

- Dry skin - this is medically termed as xeroderma. This is due to lack of water on the epidermis. As one ages too, the amount of natural oils and lubricants also diminish which lead to dry skin. The body parts prone to dryness are the arms, elbows, knees, and the lower legs. Aside from ageing, the other causes of dry skin are harsh soaps and other skin products, extreme weather, poor water intake and hot showers.

- Oily skin – the body produces natural oils. For some reasons, some people produce more body oil than what is needed. The following are the possible causes of your oily skin: genes (it runs in your family), overuse of skin products, weather conditions, some drugs, and stress. Oily skin causes acne and skin breakouts. Toners, cleansers, blotting papers and medicated pads are used to manage excessive oily skin.
- Normal skin – some people cannot distinguish if they have normal skin. That is because sometimes, the skin appears oily one time and dry the next. A normal skin has no trace of oil. It feels supple and elastic. And it has the least problem when it comes to skin conditions.
- Combination–this is common and in the face, it could be that some parts are oily (usually the nose and forehead) and some are dry, like the cheeks.

### Various skin products

Now that you are aware of the type of skin that you have, you go to the next step. Determine which product your skin needs. You are already aware that your skin's primary need is hydration. There are different hydration elements. The two most common are humectant and lubricant.

- Humectant –these retain or preserve the moisture
- Lubricant – "trap" moisture or prevent it from escaping, serving as a barrier to the skin

While both lotions and moisturizers possess these elements, not all products containing these would automatically make your skin healthy. Lotions are less viscous, meaning they are more fluid-like and thinner. They have lighter consistency. This is why they are usually in a container where you can pump it. Lotions can retain moisture that is already within the skin but not as much. They have less oil content so they do not lubricate well. For normal skin, these products would suffice.

However, for drier skin, you would need added protection and moisture-retaining products. For those individuals who have extra-dry skin, even the strongest lotion would not be enough to combat the dryness. You might want to consider trying body butters.

Know more about this skin wonder product as you read on.

# Chapter 3 Discovering Body Butters

## Discovering Body Butters

### *What are body butters?*

You may not be aware of body butters. These are actually moisturizers that contain lubricating ingredients. They are technically like lotions, only better. These ingredients serve as a protective barrier or a shield so that moisture would stay within the skin and outside environmental elements that may be harmful to the skin would not be able to come in.

Body butters are more emollient, have high viscosity and more effective for those with dry skin. Some examples of these lubricating ingredients are shea butter, coconut oil, olive and jojoba oils. Consumers also describe body butters as ensuring a "more luxurious" feel on their skin.

Body butters are extra moisturizing because they contain less water and have more essential oils or butters needed by the body to maintain moisture. Viscosity and consistency are greater so these butters are placed in jars where they would be scooped, because it would be difficult to pump them out.

Another wonder of body butter is it is ideal for those with sensitive skin. Allergies or rashes seldom occur because the ingredients of body butters are all-natural. Usually, a body butter is made up of an oil base and a few more ingredients. You would appreciate the fact that they are free from various chemicals and preservatives that could harm your skin.

## Body Lotion vs. Body Butter

Body lotion and body butter are the two most commonly used skin moisturizers. While both of them are effective in keeping your skin radiant and soft, these two products have their own unique qualities and features. In order to protect your skin better, you need to know the difference between the two moisturizers.

Lotions

Products that are identified as lotions have a lighter consistency compared to body butters. They also have very low oil percentage, and they cannot lubricate the skin. This one can accommodate every type of skin available. Lotions are also considered as humectants because they are effective at preserving the existing moisture in the body. These products usually contain alpha hydroxyl as well as hyaluronic acid. These are powerful substances that can remove dead cells from the upper layers of the skin, draw out the natural waters found in the dermis, and then send it to the epidermis.

Body lotions are highly recommended products for the hot summer months because these can keep you moisturized without making your skin too sticky and greasy. However, their light consistency does not make them ideal products for people who have dry skin.

Body Butters

Moisturizers that are considered as butters tend to be a little bit denser and highly emollient. These products are occlusive, which means that they create a protective coating on the skin. This special coat is like a barrier that defends your skin against external aggressors such as dust particles and harmful UV rays. In addition, it also helps retain moisture in your body for a long period of time. Body butter is highly recommended for people who have extremely dry skin because these are thicker and more viscous than creams and lotions.

Aside from acting as a moisturizer, body butter also helps rejuvenate your skin, reduce the wrinkles or visible lines on your face, and make you look extremely younger. This is an ideal product during the cold winter months because it keeps your skin moisturized for a long period of time.

If you have oily skin, it is not recommended that you use body butter all the time. The protective barrier that it creates tends to block out your pores, thus making your skin a good breeding ground for bacteria.

**Different Uses of Body Butter**

Aside from being a moisturizing agent, body butter can actually be used in several different ways. Check these out below:

1.  Hand Care – you can use body butter to keep your hands soft. You just need to apply small amounts of this product every day so that your fingers will stay moisturized all the time. If your hands are quite dry, apply large quantities of it before you go to bed. For better results, you can also put on a pair of cotton gloves while you sleep.
2.  Smoothing out Dry Patches – if you have flaky elbows or toes, then this product is perfect for you. All you have to do is apply small quantities of body butter on

the dry regions of your skin. Afterwards, massage it a little bit so that it can easily be absorbed by the body.

3. Foot Care – After thoroughly washing your feet, massage them with body butter on a daily basis to them supple and soft. It is also recommended that you apply large amounts of this product on your feet, cover them with cotton socks overnight. This simple treatment can rejuvenate your skin quickly.

4. Cuticle Softener – slather some of this butter on your fingers and toes to make it easier for you to remove your cuticles.

5. Eye Makeup Remover – roll a dampened cotton ball on a piece of body butter. Then, lightly scrub off the makeup. This can also be used to remove water-proof mascara, as well as maintaining the beauty of your eyelashes.

6. Face moisturizer – Work a small amount of body butter on your hands before applying it. Afterwards, lightly massage your face using upward strokes. Stroke your palms across your forehead. Then, slightly pinch your jaw line. Finally, apply using upward strokes on your cheeks. Regularly massaging your face will surely remove your wrinkles and fine lines.

7. Décolletage Moisturizer – smear some of the butter on your neck. Use upward strokes to massage your neck. Repeat this process on a daily basis.

8. Aftershave and leg balm – body butter also removes the "fish scales" that you acquire after shaving.

9. Lip Balm – Apply this product similar to how you do it with other types of lip balm.

10. Massage – Had an extremely stressful day? Body butter offers a soothing and relaxing feeling to your body too.

Do you want to know another wonder of body butters? You could actually make your own body butters right in the comfort of your home. They are easy to make and the ingredients are not that hard to find.

Are you ready for a healthier skin? Find out more about making your own body butters.

# Chapter 4 Beauty Within Your Reach

## Beauty Within Your Reach

It is time to end the confusion on which products suit you. It is time to make your own body butters.

One great thing about body butters is the availability of the ingredients. You could avail a lot of these even from your local stores. You would notice though that the ingredients are mostly derived from nuts and seeds. So if you are allergic to these types of food, it is wise to consult your primary health care provider first just to be sure if topical applications would be hazardous to you.

Here are some of the basic ingredients of body butter.

1. Cocoa butter – Cocoa butter is made from cocoa beans. Cocoa beans come from the fleshy cocoa fruits. After cleaning and roasting, the beans are placed in a machine where the cocoa butter would be produced. Of course, in your local store, you could just buy it as a cocoa butter already. This is actually a vegetable fat that is edible. It is used mostly for making chocolates and beauty products. What makes this as a good ingredient to help your skin? The cocoa itself contains large amounts of antioxidants called flavonoids. It is also rich in potassium, calcium and iron. These allow veins to be more relaxed. This promotes good circulation and at the same time, help fight against free radicals that are harmful to the body. Not to mention, this smells good too.

2. Shea butter – Another common ingredient of body butter is shea butter. This comes from the nut of the African shea tree or karite tree. This is also known as karite butter. Like the cocoa butter, this extracted fat is also edible and can be used in making chocolates. This ingredient has been known to be very effective in the fight against stretch marks. It has been internationally recognized to treat various skin disorders as well. This is because it has been found to contain anti-inflammatory properties. It is also an anti-ageing agent. The vitamins found in shea butter help in preventing the occurrence of wrinkles and other facial lines. Plus it can be a form of sunblock and even as a relief for nasal congestion and sinusitis.

3. Coconut oil – Much has been written about the wonders of this ingredient. In some tropical areas, the coconut tree is considered as the tree of life. It has been used for thousands of years not only as skin beautifier but as supplements to help conquer Alzheimer disease, Diabetes Mellitus, Thyroid problems, weight concerns and even hair problems like lice and dandruff. Coconut is known to be the number one source of lauric acids. These acids have been known to fight off pathogens or harmful organisms in the body.

4. Mango butter – Another great ingredient is mango butter which is an oil extracted from the kernel of a mango. It has anti-inflammatory, anti-oxidant and anti-ageing properties, making it a favorite among

cosmetics suppliers. It contains oleic and stearic acids in very large amounts. These make mango butter highly emollient and thus ideal in sealing moisture within the body. It highly nourishes the skin, too. Plus it has a very sweet and refreshing smell. Mango butter can also provide protection from the sun. It also non-greasy and very soothing to touch.

5. Cinnamon – The common kitchen ingredient cinnamon has some uncommon qualities. Do you know that it is a proven antimicrobial, anti-fungal and antibacterial agent? What's more, it has an astringent property, which helps make the skin firmer and clearer as it removes blemishes. Cinnamon is gaining popularity because it is also very rich in magnesium, iron and calcium. These are minerals that help keep skin healthy. Cinnamon is great for body butters as it also helps local blood circulation. A good circulation allows for delivery of nutrients and oxygen to the different parts of the body. This has been used in the fight against acne and has shown to remove impurities and to aid as an anti inflammatory substance as well.

6. Honey – Raw honey is a humectant. It helps retain water so that the skin is kept moisturized. Honey as a cosmetic agent has been used for thousands of years already. It was discovered to contain skin restorative properties. Just a little amount can go a long way in making the skin youthful looking. Honey also contains

germ-fighting bacteria, which help in fighting off the enemies of the skin.

7. Other ingredients – do not be surprise that other nuts and seeds can be included as ingredients too in any body butter that you could make. As long as there is the base oil or lubricant, you could add other ingredients that could enhance the feel, the smell and the color of the body butter. These are peppermint, rosemary, lavender, magnesium, black raspberry, coffee, cinnamon, vanilla, lemon, avocado and the list goes on.

You can enjoy tremendous peace of mind since you are 100% sure that what you are using won't harm your skin or make it look unsightly. With these ingredients, you could start making your own body butter now. Plus it can also be a great gift idea for your family and friends.

Having healthy skin need not be difficult nor expensive. Start having great skin that you could show off! Start making your own body butters.

# Chapter 5  Simple Recipes For A Great Skin

### Simple Recipes For Great Skin

Do you know that you can make as many as one hundred or more different body butters for your skin? That's right, and all these at the comfort of your own home with no special machinery needed. You do not even have to be a chef to do these. You could be a beginner and a master at making body butters at the same time.

Here are simple tips before you start.

1. Remember to check if you have any allergic reaction or even sensitivity to any of the ingredients that you are going to use. If unsure, it is better to try it out on a small portion of your arm first. If you cannot spot any allergic reactions, such as itchiness, redness, warm feeling or any sign of irritation, then you can try it on other parts until you have proven that it is safe for you.

2. Melting the oils is one basic action in making your own body butter. Try to melt it slowly by using low to medium level of heat. Do not place the oil at a high level of heat at any time.

3. You would also be asked to chill or set the oil. This is allowing the oils to cool and then form into a semi-solid state. If you would set it in a room temperature, it could take hours. In the refrigerator, estimated time for the oils to set is 15-20 minutes.  Chilling properly is important because you would not want it to be

frozen. It could kill some of the vitamins and minerals on the oils, rendering it useless. And you would also have difficulty in getting the right viscosity of the body butter.

4. Finally, you would be asked to whip it until it reaches the butter-like consistency.

The body butters should be placed on clean glass jars.

The finished product should be maintained at a cool temperature to keep it from melting. But if it does melt, simply stir or whip it again until it returns to its previous consistency.

The homemade product's lifespan depends on many factors. This includes the humidity of the storage area, the ingredients that you used, cooking methods, types of jar that you used, and a whole lot more. If you have properly prepared the body butter, it can last for a couple of months.

But to be on the safe side, try to use it for three months at the most. There are reports of 6 months up to a year of useful life for these products.

### *Cooking Time*

It is time to start making those body butters. Here are some of the most highly recommended simple recipes that you can try out.

1. Triple delight body butter – Simply melt 1 cup shea butter and ½ cup coconut oil in the top of a double boiler. Once melted, allow the mixture to cool for 30 minutes. Stir in the half cup of almond oil. Place in the freezer or chiller (this is very important – chilling should just be right. It is about 20 minutes). Whip

into a butter-like consistency when the oil starts to partially become solid. Place in a clean jar and then use for hydrating and rejuvenating your skin. Keep in a cool place. Simple right?

2. Vanilla Secret Body Butter – Do you know that vanilla can serve as aphrodisiac? Feel sexier as you use this body butter. Melt a cup of cocoa butter and half cup of coconut oil. Remove from heat and allow to cool for thirty minutes. While waiting to cool, grind in a coffee grinder (or you could also use a food processor) a single vanilla bean. Place in a container. Stir in half cup of sweet almond oil into the vanilla bits plus the cooled oil mixture. Place in a freezer to chill. Wait until the oils start to be partially solid. Then using an electric mixer or a food processor, whip until it becomes like butter. There you have a vanilla body butter, which you could use to attract your partner too.

3. Mango & Shea Body Butter - Combine the following ingredients in a double boiler – ½ cup shea butter, ½ cup mango butter, ½ cup coconut oil and ½ cup olive or jojoba. Constantly stir as you melt all the oils. Remove from heat and allow to cool for 30 minutes. Place in the freezer until it starts to harden but it is still soft. Whip until fluffy and there you have it! Your own body butter for a more beautiful skin!

4. Rose Scented Coconut body butter – As you melt, cool and place the cup of coconut oil in the freezer, just add a few drops of rose scented oil to perfect the moisturizer. When in a semi solid stage, whip until it becomes butter-like in consistency. You would not only have a soft skin but you would simply adore that perfume like smell.

5. No-cook body butter – place all the ingredients in a food processor or blender. These are ¾ cup melted coconut oil, ½ tablespoons vanilla powder, ¼ cup cacao powder and 1/3 cup clear agave. Blend and then place them in clean glass or jars and then place in the refrigerator to set in.

6. Fruity body butter – combine half cup each of cocoa and shea butters. Melt and allow to cool. Add around 10-20 drops (depends on how fruity you like it to smell) of Black Raspberry Fragrance Oil. Place in the refrigerator to set it. Once it is almost solid, whip it until it becomes like butter in consistency. You will then have a body butter that smells so cool.

7. Lemony Body Butters – Place 6 tablespoons coconut oil and ¼ cup cacao butter in a saucepan and melt it. Remove from heat and add 1 teaspoon lemon essential oil. Cool until the mixture solidifies. Whip and it is ready to use. You would love its refreshing lemon smell.

8. Pretty in Pink Body butter – this is a great idea for a gift. It looks charming with its pink color too. Melt 6 ounces coconut oil and 2 ounces cocoa butter in a low heat double boiler. After melting, remove from heat and let it cool. You could make this faster by placing it in the refrigerator. Once it is partially solid, you can whip this manually or use an electric mixer. The oils would turn creamy. Place this creamy oil in the refrigerator again for five minutes and then whip again. At this point, you could add essential oil like rosemary or peppermint until you get stiff peaks. As it is, it is already attractive and healthy for your skin. However, you could make it daintier by adding red

colorant to the finished product, giving it a pinkish shade.

9.  Glowing Skin Body Butter – the secret to this recipe is the use of extra virgin, raw and organic coconut oil. The feel afterwards is extra smooth and soft skin. Like the other recipes, just add this special 2 cups of coconut oil and 7 ounces of shea butter and allow to melt in a saucepan. Cool and at this time, you could add a drop of tea tree oil. Tea tree oil is known for its antimicrobial and antibacterial properties. You could also add any essential oils that you like. Peppermint, jasmine or rosemary smells great on this combination. This is optional though. Cool, set in and then whip. You now have a body butter that is sure to make your skin healthier and softer.

10. Cinnamon Power Packed Body Butter – Melt 50 grams cocoa butter and 50 grams shea butter until it becomes a liquid. Add 100 grams coconut oil, stir in gently for a minute and then remove the oils from heat. Let it cool for 30 minutes. Add 30 drops of cinnamon oil as soon as it cools. Then whip until it becomes fluffy and butter-like. Before pouring it to containers, add some bits of cinnamon stick on it. Preferable containers are airtight.

That was easy, right? Even a first timer would get it right. You could do some mixing and matching of ingredients and you could even invent your own body butter. Make your own until you find the one that suits you perfectly. You would know if it is the perfect one for you when your skin feels so soft and smooth. You would also notice that your skin looks hydrated. This is because the moisture is locked in.

It is also recommended that you try and change the skin products every six months. This is to have a variety of available minerals and vitamins for your skin. Changing your body butters would also allow you to enjoy different smells and effects on your skin.

# Chapter 6 More Tips For A Healthier Skin

### More Tips For A Healthier Skin

Healthy Radiant Skin

Body butters and other moisturizers are big help when it comes to rejuvenated and hydrated skin. However, there are other things you could do to ensure a healthier skin.

### *Basic care for the skin*

Caring for the skin cannot be overemphasized. Here are some simple things you can do to care for your skin.

1. Clean according to skin type. Different skin types require different kind of cleaning. For dry skin, use a mild cleansing product and clean only once, preferably at night. For oily skin, you could wash and clean it twice in a day. For the combination type, combine also the style of cleansing. For normal skin, regular washing would do. Follow the instructions on the labels of the products carefully.
2. Remove all make up. As much as possible, allow your skin to rest by not wearing any make up. If you do need to wear makeup, make sure that you totally remove it at the end of the day by washing thoroughly. Pat dry.
3. Protection from the sun. Your skin's number one enemy is the sun, although the sun is a friend from 7-8am. Afterwards, try to avoid its harmful rays as

much as possible. You could apply sunscreen, use umbrella or wear clothes with sleeves.

4. Exfoliate. This simply means to remove the dead skin (you have millions of them remember?). You could do this on skin without breaks. There are products available in your local grocery store for exfoliation. Follow the instructions very well.

5. Water. When you think of skin, you want it to be hydrated at all times. By simply drinking 8-10 glasses a day, you are already helping your skin to be hydrated and radiant.

6. Do not scratch, pick on pimples, remove scabs or do anything that would break the skin. Keep it intact at all cost. You should also try to trim your nails so that they would not cause damage to your skin.

7. Supplements to help. Aside from eating healthy foods like fruits and vegetables, vitamins a, b, c and e can also help skin become healthier, softer and more beautiful.

8. Healthy lifestyle. Drinking alcoholic beverages, sleeping late, smoking, and eating junk foods are just some of the way that would harm your skin. Try having healthy habits and get enough rest and sleep.

9. Lotions and other products. To keep your skin from drying or just to moisturize it, there are various products that you can choose from and use. Find which one suits you best. Extreme weathers would require that you use these products more often to protect your skin.

*Prevent your skin from aging rapidly*

At some point in your life, you will become old, and you will have wrinkles. When you age, your skin will lose its ability to heal itself faster. Exposure to UV rays, the facial expressions you make, your current lifestyle habits, and even the earth's gravitational pull can greatly affect your skin, and not in a good way. That is a fact of life that cannot be prevented.

However, that good news is that there are numerous methods that you can try to prolong the natural beauty of your skin. Below is a list of healthy habits that you should try if you want to maintain a youthful appearance.

1. Use sunscreen. This is one of the simplest yet most often neglected tricks in the skin care bible. Sunscreen is one of the best topical products that you can use to protect yourself against the harmful UV rays of the sun. Although it does not fix the fine lines on your skin, it prevents the skin from being damaged by the sun's UV rays. Keep in mind that sunscreen is not a magic beauty product that will make you look beautiful once you apply it. Unlike other anti-aging products, it may take years before you finally the benefits of using sunscreen. If you do not want to use sunscreen, you can also opt to wear hats to protect your skin when you go outdoors. In addition, do not stay in the sun for too long during its peak hours.

2. Eat proper nutrients. You are what you eat. It might sound a little bit cliché, but it is true. If you eat foods that are rich in vitamins C, E, and A, you will have an extremely healthy skin. Eating five to seven servings of carrots, citrus fruits, or tomatoes every day will surely make you look younger.

3. Do regular exercise. Aside from improving your overall health and well-being, doing regular exercise

can actually provide a lot of benefits for your skin. Physical exercises improve the circulation of your blood. This means that your skin cells will be properly nourished, and their harmful free radicals will be removed. However, make sure that you exercise inside a gym or in your house so that your skin will not be exposed to sunlight.

4. Relax. As much as possible, do not put yourself in extremely stressful situations. When you are under pressure, your body produces cortisol, a hormone that can ravage your collagen. This will then prevent your skin from repairing itself quickly. Stress can also force you to frown. Excessive frowning on a regular basis will definitely leave a permanent mark on your face. To relieve stress, you should do a little bit of yoga or Tai Chi. Brisk walking can also be beneficial because it relaxes your mind while you do it.

5. Use cleansers. Try a gentle cleanser that can effectively remove dirt without destroying your protective layer of oil and moisture. Products with alpha-hydroxy acids, more commonly known as AHAs, are beneficial for exfoliating your dead skin cells and making your skin glow.

6. Wash yourself thoroughly after taking a dip in the pool. Swimming pools are filled with chlorine – a chemical that can make your skin hair and dry. Chlorine is a stubborn compound that can cling tightly to your skin. Do not attempt to use topical medications and cleansers to remove it because it reacts with these products and might produce

irritations and rashes. In order to completely remove chlorine, use a super sudsy soap after you take a swim.

7. Never go to sleep with your make-up on. This will promote the growth of harmful bacteria on your skin. In addition, it will clog your pores, thus, causing acne. Any make-up residue that is left on your pillow can also cause you to be sick. Make it a habit to remove your mascara or eyeliner before you hit the sack.

8. Do not wax too often. You may not have a passion for unwanted facial hairs, but if you want to have youthful-looking skin, do not wax too often. Excessive waxing will make your skin raw. After you have removed your facial hairs, allow your skin cells to regenerate for at least three weeks or more before attempting another waxing session.

A healthy skin is a goal that everybody must have. Skin care is easy and the rewards are awesome. Hydrated and rejuvenated skin looks great and at the same time, it is a great protector of the body. Enjoy a smooth and flawless skin now!

# Chapter 7 – Setting up your Own Body Butter Shop

Now that you know how to cook your very own body butter recipes, you may want to think about starting your very own bath and body business. Not only can you gain extra profit from your skills, you can also help other women have vibrant and supple skin.

A lot of people are now enticed to use natural beauty products because of their positive side effects on the body. Since the industry is booming these days, it means that you will never run out of customers.

Setting up your own shop may seem like a very daunting task, but in reality, it is actually pretty easy and fun. With a little bit of hard work, creativity, and passion, you may even see your products displayed on the shelves of retail outlets in your area and possibly beyond.

If you are interested in this endeavor, here are some basic guidelines to help you get started in your new bath and body business.

**Factors to Consider**

**1. Supply of natural ingredients**
As a seller of homemade body butter, your biggest advantage against sellers of other bath and body products on the market is that you only use natural ingredients. This makes your body butter safer to use.

If you are serious about entering this industry, you need to have access to a vast supply of natural ingredients such as mint leaves, cinnamon, cocoa, peppermint, coconut oil, and other vital items for your recipe.

You can have these ingredients for free if you plant them in your backyard. However, not everyone has a lot of extra gardening space. If that is true in your case, then you can purchase these items from specialty shops and suppliers.

## 2. Equipment

The good thing about making your own body butter is that you do not need a lot of expensive tools.

Most of the tools that you will need for concocting your bath and body products are found in your very own kitchen. A basic body butter kit should have cooking pots, pans, food mixer, mixing bowl, and other basic cooking utensils.

For storing the body butter, you need to acquire glass jars or small plastic tubs. Depending on the number of customers that you have, you need to purchase these containers in bulk. Do not worry about the costs because you can easily find cheap prices for these items.

You can easily purchase secondhand glass jars in auctions, garage sales, and even warehouse sales. However, make sure that they are free from any nicks and cracks. For hygienic and sanitary purposes, make sure that you buy a new lid for every glass jar that you bought.

You may also need a little bit of arts and crafts materials. Part of starting a bath and body business is the packaging of your products. Of course, you do not want to sell your body butter in cheap looking containers, do you? You need to add a little bit of sizzle to your products by incorporating appropriate designs on their containers. As an owner of a flourishing business, you have the freedom to go crazy with the designs. Just make sure that the designs are unique enough to be popular among your customers.

## 3. New Skills

Aside from learning how to cook the body butter, you also need to learn a couple of new skills in order to make your business flourish.

You need to learn how to properly preserve and contain your products. Body butter needs to be a little bit soft. Body butter is a little bit tricky to handle because if you do not cook it right, it might be less viscous and thick. In addition, you also need to store it in a room with the temperature and level of humidity so that its texture will remain constant. If you are still not adept at doing this, you can take up extra classes regarding this subject.

Another skill that you should acquire is marketing. During the early stages of your bath and body business, you may have to do these marketing tasks on your own. Thankfully, there are various tools that you can use in this endeavor.

## Marketing Tips for Newbie Bath and Body Entrepreneurs

The quality of the product is not enough to help you earn a lot of profit. You also need to use several marketing techniques in order to sell your product.

As an independent seller of bath and body products, you may not have the adequate financial resources to market your items via traditional media such as television commercials, or print advertisements. However, that does not mean that you cannot pull off a winning strategy on a tight budget. The list below shows some of the simplest yet most highly effective marketing techniques that you can use for your business endeavors.

## 1. Utilize social media tools

Aside from playing online games and catching up with your friends, you can also use social media platforms to increase other people's awareness about your products.

A great example of this one is Pinterest. This one is a social media platform that allows its users to easily share and "pin" photographs on their virtual boards. These pictures could then be seen by their friends and followers. You can take this to your advantage by sharing your amazing body butter recipes.

When it comes to using social media networks, it is highly recommended that you spread yourself across various platforms. Aside from Facebook, you should also create your Twitter and Google+ profiles. However, keep in mind that each social media platform has its own strengths and weaknesses. You need to understand all of their features so that you can tailor the right content for them.

Another important social media tip that you should learn is to post relevant content that your target market appreciates. Since you are running a bath and body business, you should regularly post some information about beauty tips, skin care, advantages of using natural products, and a whole lot more. You can grab articles and blog posts from other websites, or, you can create your own written pieces.

Aside from articles, you can also post some videos and pictures about bath and body topics. You need to mix up the content so that your followers will be enticed to visit your pages all the time.

In addition, it is also important that you interact with your friends and followers on a regular basis. Make sure that you answer their inquiries, especially if these inquiries are about your products.

## 2. Host an Event

Hosting an event can help increase your popularity in the community. You can create body butter seminars, or team up with your local spa and create a special massage event using your body butter. Make sure that the event that you will host is in line with the products that you sell so that it will be totally effective.

If you have set up your own store, it is ideal that you set the event in that place so that people will discover its location.

## 3. Support fundraising activities

This marketing strategy will help establish a good reputation for your brand. You can donate money, some of your selected products, and even your services to these fundraising activities.

However, keep in mind that the charity event that you will join should be related to the products that you sell. Mentioning the name of your brand during these events will greatly help you become known to the public. However, it is best if you can also showcase your products.

If you are supporting a fun run, maybe you can provide free samples of your body butter. They can apply your product on their face and hands before the race starts. That way, the people will discover the quality of your body butter and its amazing benefits to their skin.

In addition, be sure that your target market will also be attending the event.

## 4. Join local clubs

As an entrepreneur, it is vital that you make yourself more visible, especially if you own a physical shop instead of an online one. If you have any local business clubs, join them if possible. You can meet a lot of influential people in these organizations. You can do business partnerships with them, and they can help promote your body butter products. Some clubs even request their members to give public speeches and seminars.

## 5. Develop a Website for your Body Butter Business

A lot of people tend to do their shopping online, so it is ideal if you build a website to handle these customers. Buying a website domain can be extremely cheap, so you will not have to worry about exceeding your marketing budget. You have the freedom to design it yourself, or you can outsource it. With articles and blog posts, your online presence will be further increased.

# Chapter 8 –Massage your Body Using Body Butter

Aside from being an effective moisturizer for dry skin, you can also apply natural butter on your body to have a pleasing massage experience. Most types of body butter, especially the ones that are infused with cocoa or mint leaves, can have a very soothing aroma that can eradicate the stress that you acquired during the day.

Massaging your body also has great benefits for your body. First of all, it improves blood circulation in certain areas such as your face, shoulders, and neck. That way, essential nutrients will be evenly distributed across these parts. It lubricates your joints so that it will not be prone to medical conditions like arthritis and rheumatism. Furthermore, doing regular self-massage therapy can also calm your nerves and help promote a positive outlook in life. If you find it hard to sleep, these relaxation techniques can be used to help cure your insomnia.

Here is a list of simple self-massage techniques that you can do if you want to relax your mind and body. Feel free to use any body butter that you prefer for each type of massage.

### Therapy for Relaxing the Hands
Are your hands too stiff and tired from pounding the keyboard all day? Try stretching them a little bit every once in a while. Hands have certain reflexology points that correspond with your different body parts. This means that if you massage your hands, your head, neck, sinuses, eyes, and

other parts of the body will be relaxed as well. Here's how you can do it:

1. Extend your hands and fingers. Rub each of your digits from top to bottom. Lightly pull and twist your fingers while rubbing them.
2. Place your left hand on your lap. Its palm should be facing upward.
3. Gently squeeze the soft spot located in the middle of your thumb and index finger.
4. Rub the rest of the palm using your right thumb. Apply firm pressure as your thumb glides across the wrist to your left hand's fingers.
5. Repeat this massage routine on your right hand.

**Reducing Tension in your Neck Area**

1. While sitting in your chair, cast your hands over your shoulders. Breathe deeply and allow your head to slightly drop back.
2. Gently move your fingers to your palms, while letting the muscles on your shoulders slide to your neck.
3. Slightly drop your head forward by placing your elbows on the table.
4. Using your fingertips, massage your neck, shoulders, and the bottom of your skull by drawing deep, yet small circles on your spine.
5. Put both of your hands on your head's backside. Make sure that your fingers are interlaced with each other. Let your head drop forward while feeling the weight of your elbows.

**Relaxing Massage for your Tired Feet**

Simple tasks such as jogging or shopping for groceries can put a lot of strain on your feet. After several hours of walking around, your feet might start to ache. If you do not rest your tired soles, it might impair your walking for life. Although most people prefer to use special types of shoes to fix this problem, nothing can beat a good old foot massage to soothe away the pain. Here is how you can do it:

1. Raise your left foot on your chair so that you can easily see your instep.
2. Use your right thumb to slowly apply firm pressure on the sides of your foot. Start running your thumb on your heels and slowly work your way towards your big toe.
3. Run your thumb on the ridge that connects your toes and your metatarsalgia (also known as the ball of your foot).
4. Once you small toe, squeeze its surface using your thumb and index fingers.
5. Grab all the toes on your left foot and then stretch them out back and forth.
6. Hold the tip of your foot using your left hand.
7. Using your other hand's knuckles, apply firm pressure on the entire sole of your feet.
8. Stretch out your toes, and do several ankle rotations.
9. Repeat the process on the other foot.

**Shiatsu Facial Massage**

Geishas were revered across the various parts of Japan because of their very smooth and beautiful face. Another amazing thing about these performers is that even though some of them were old, they managed to maintain such youthful appearances.

The secret to their unfading beauty is that they use the Shiatsu massage technique. They did this facial therapy on a daily basis, so they maintained their attractive appearance. This massage is all about applying light touches on your face using your fingertips. The good thing about this therapy is that it will not consume too much of your time; it will only take you five minutes to do it.

1. Locate the pressure point on your temples. You can tell that it is a pressure point because of the slight pain that you will feel when you touch it. Using your fingertips, massage the pressure points using a circular motion. Repeat this step for three times.
2. Close your eyes. Slowly press your fingers on the inner corners of your eyelids. Do this process for three times.
3. Use the palm of your hand, massage your neck. Start from the base near the shoulders up. Then, slowly move your way towards the neck's top near the jaws.
4. Firmly press your middle and index finger on top of your forehead. Massage its middle part, and then slowly move towards your temples. This will help smoothen out the lines in your forehead.
5. Start applying pressure on the corners of your mouth. Begin the therapy on your lower lip. Then, massage the outer corners of your mouth.
6. Massage your cheeks using your fingertips. Apply firm pressure while moving your fingers in a circular motion.

**Su-Man's Special Facial Massage**

Su-Man is a popular celebrity facial specialist who is known for her pioneering skin treatment that combines the oriental facial massage, and the elements of shiatsu.

It is highly recommended that you repeat every massage stroke for 36 times. According to popular Chinese belief, six is a very lucky number that will help a person achieve optimal health conditions, happiness, and of course, a younger-looking skin.

Su-Man's special facial massage should be done after cleaning your face. Make sure that you only touch the parts of your face using clean hands.

1.  Generate adequate amount of heat on your face by rubbing your ears using the palm of your hands.
2.  Rest your elbows on a smooth table.
3.  Start massaging your chin using the heels of your palms. Slowly move towards the base of your ears.
4.  Using the heels of your palms again, stroke the edge of your nostrils. Keep applying pressure until you reach your cheekbones.
5.  Use your index and middle fingers and apply some pressure on the sides of your eyes and nose. You need to follow your nose line and firmly stroke in a downwards direction. Aside from making you look more beautiful, this is also beneficial for clearing up your sinus and improve your breathing.
6.  Shape little claws using four fingers from each of your hands. Place them in the middle region of your forehead.

7. Press that area firmly, but make sure that you do not puncture your skin. Squeeze your forehead in an upward direction. Then, do the same on your temples.

8. Close your eyes and slightly tap your eye sockets. Stroke six times above the sockets and six times below it. This simple activity is helpful in brightening your eyes, as well as minimizing the puffiness below your eyes.

# Chapter 9 – Preserving Bath and Body Products

Just like food, body butters can also become spoiled and rotten in the long run. If you do not preserve and store it properly, it might do more harm on your face and overall health.

Body butters can harbor bacteria, yeast, and molds when they are not used for a long period of time. Since you have skipped some of the processes that the large manufacturers have done in order to improve the shelf life of their beauty products, expect that your body butter will rot faster. To help you out, here are some simple yet effective tips in prolonging the shelf life of your homemade body butters.

## 1. Clean your hands and disinfect all your tools before using them

Spoilage can be prevented if you can remove all the germs in your hands and cooking equipment.

Before you begin cooking your homemade beauty products, you must disinfect your hands and cooking utensils so that no harmful molds, bacteria, yeast, will contaminate the finished product. So clean your hands with soap and water, sanitize your kitchen, spatula, bottles, mixing bowl, and other vital items that you will use for cooking. In order to pull this off, you can opt to soak the equipment in hot water. If their surfaces are dirty, scrub them off with a sponge and dishwashing liquid. Rinse thoroughly so that no soap residue will be left on the utensils.

Afterwards, you need to make sure that the items are totally dry. To make this process quicker, use a paper towel, or a clean soft rag to wipe off their surfaces. Most unwanted yeasts and molds require a lot of moisture in the environment in order to propagate. If the cooking materials and containers are still wet, these microorganisms will surely accumulate in your body butters and destroy them. Lastly, always use a small spatula or tablespoon instead of your fingers whenever you want to scoop up little quantities of the body butter's ingredients.

## 2. Only create small batches

As mentioned earlier, most beauty products that are created at home do not have any preservatives. This makes them more susceptible to spoilage than the ones that are mass-produced in factories.

If you do not want to waste your time and effort, make sure that you only concoct small batches of body butter at home. In addition, use them immediately while they are still fresh. Keep in mind that body butter contains liquids, so expect that they will rot sooner than other dry beauty products such as bath soaps and bath bombs.

If there is some excess body butter, just give them away to your friends or family so that they can be consumed quickly.

## 3. Use preservatives if you are making an exceptionally bigger batch

But if you are running a small business and you really needed to produce large quantities of body butter, the best course to take is to use preservatives.

For this problem, you can opt to use synergistic preservatives. This product is the offspring of various types of preservatives that were combined together. They are created to kill bacteria, mold and fungi by causing a chemical disruption in their environment. These products are highly effective for liquid products such as lotions, moisturizers, and body butter.

There are also natural preservatives that you can use in order to prolong the shelf life of your body butter. An example of this one is Vitamin E. Technically, it is not really a preservative per se, but rather, it is an antioxidant. Thanks to this feature, Vitamin E can slow down the rate of oxidation in your body butter, thus prolonging its shelf life for a little bit. Aside from preserving the product, it will also improve the product's effectiveness.

Another great alternative is to use essential oils that contain antimicrobial properties. Examples of these oils include grapefruit seed, rosemary, lavender, and sage. These ingredients are powerful enough to fend off any harmful bacteria, yeast, and mold that might accumulate in your body butters.

The downside of using this product is that you need to use large quantities in order to make them work. Too much oil in your body butter will affect its consistency. Moreover, you need to have adequate knowledge when it comes to infusing oils in cosmetic products. Chemists who are adept at making cosmetic products have a specific formula when it comes to mixing essential oils with beauty products. If you are not knowledgeable about it, you may produce a body butter that is harmful to your skin. Before you use any lavender or thyme oil, make sure that the recipe that you are following clearly stated the exact amount of oil that you should use.

## 4. Observe proper storage methods

Body butter, and other types of cosmetic products, has the tendency to lose their effectiveness once they are exposed to light or air. To preserve their soothing and moisturizing properties, always use a container that is opaque and totally air tight. Since homemade products contain little or no amount of preservatives, it is highly recommended if you put them in tubes or dispensing jars. This will ensure that no bacteria can penetrate your products. When not in use, store them in a cool and dry place such as your cabinet, cupboard, and even your refrigerator. Do not use your hands when the body butter because the germs from your fingers might contaminate the rest of the products inside the container. Instead, use a clean spatula.

## 5. If you smell something funny in your ingredients, do not use it

If you notice that your fruits and oils give off a very pungent scent, avoid using these products anymore because they might be spoiled.

Unlike cooking meals, you can still salvage some parts of a spoiled fruit by turning them into puree or jelly. However, you can use the same technique with cosmetic products. The bacteria and other harmful elements might still be alive in these ingredients. If you still use them to create body butter, they might negatively affect the finished product. If you want

49

your face to look fresh, you have to make sure that you only use the freshest ingredients available.

## 6. Use antimicrobials

Antimicrobials are effective agents that can destroy any unwanted fungi and bacteria hiding inside your body butter. Examples of natural antimicrobials include:

- **Coconut oil** – it is replete with lauric acid and caprylic acid. These are two powerful acids that have the ability to prevent fungi from spreading in your products.

- **Grapefruit seed extracts** – This is one of the most common natural preservatives that are found in beauty products such as bar soaps, moisturizers, and lotions. The grape seed extract ratio that you should use is 0.5 – 1% per batch.

- **Other essential oils** – This includes cumin, caraway, sandalwood, and eucalyptus. Make sure that you only use small amounts of these ingredients in order to prevent any negative skin reactions.

**Factors to consider when using preservatives**
Before picking the right preservative for your body butter, you need to consider several factors first. This is to ensure that your product will be completely effective and your skin will be safe from any unwanted chemical reactions. Here are

some of the things that you should consider when choosing an appropriate preservative.

1. What are the kinds of ingredients that you are using? Are they soluble in oil, or are they soluble in water?
2. What is the final pH of the finished product? Keep in mind that you do not want to make your body butter become too acidic.
3. What type of container are you using?
4. Will the preservatives last for a long period of time?
5. Can they work under less favorable conditions? What if the body butter accidentally gets exposed to light? Can it effectively eliminate any potential dangers that might befall on my product?
6. Will the preservatives act quickly when the body butter suddenly becomes contaminated?
7. Is it friendly to sensitive skin?
8. Are the preservatives devoid of any toxic chemicals that might further irritate the skin?
9. Will it mix well with the rest of ingredients in the formula?
10. Are the preservatives stable? Will they suddenly disintegrate when exposed to extremely hot temperatures?

# Chapter 10 – Body Butter Myths Debunked

Although body butter is already proven to be a useful product that is ideal for making your skin look more radiant and younger, most people are still skeptical about using this product.

What is worse is that a lot of them are spreading wrong information about body butters. People who are not too knowledgeable about this product will easily accept these lies and misconceptions as truths.

In addition, misinformation can also do grave harm to people who are enthusiastic about using this product. Sometimes, they practice the wrong methods when using body butter. That is why their skin does not look too radiant and youthful even though they regularly apply the product all over their body.

If you want to gain the great benefits that body butter has to offer, you need to arm yourselves with the right information. Below is a list of myths about body butter and the truth behind them.

**Myth 1: Using body butter for a single time will help my skin become smoother and more beautiful.**

This belief is totally incorrect. Just like any other beauty product, body butter is not a magical potion that can instantly make you beautiful. If at first you do not see any visible changes in your body, do not get frustrated. It might take a little while before you finally see the benefits of body butter.

The secret to making it work is to apply the product on a regular basis. If you use body butter every day, you can see visible results in no time at all.

**Myth 2: Body butter is the only thing I need in order to make myself look more radiant.**

This is another misconception that most people have when it comes to body butter. This product is highly effective because of its bevy of natural ingredients. However, there are still several factors that can greatly affect the quality of your skin. Your lifestyle, the food that you eat, and your environment can greatly affect the natural beauty of your skin.

In order to be really radiant and beautiful, you still need to start living a healthier lifestyle. This means that you have to avoid extremely oily foods, smoking, and excessive drinking. Exercise can also be beneficial for your appearance because it promotes healthy circulation of blood and nutrients to your skin cells.

You can also mix and match other cosmetic products to ensure your beautiful looks. Body butter is effective in keeping your skin moisturized all the time. However, there is also a wide array of natural bath and body products that you can try in order to protect your body. This includes soaps, lotions, oils, and a whole lot more. Make sure that you the products complement each other so that they will be more effective.

**Myth 3: You can use body butter on your hair**
Only some types of body butter can be used to treat your hair. If your product contains too much oil, you should not apply it on your scalp because it will make your strands too greasy and stiff. However, body butter that is made from Shea or coconut butter can be applied to your hair.

You can also modify your body butter so that it can be effective on your scalp too. You can ingredients such as:

- **Wax (beeswax or carnauba is highly preferred)** – This is useful for removing any frizzles on your coiled strands. In addition, it can also create a protective layer that prevents any moisture from seeping away from your skin and hair.

- **Aloe** – This natural ingredient is one of the most effective humectants that are available on the market. In addition, it is also an anti-inflammatory agent that prevents any irritations from occurring on the scalp. However, keep in mind that aloe vera is water soluble. This means that you need to use preservatives to prolong its shelf life and effectiveness. It is also highly recommended if you store it inside your refrigerator.

- **Extracts and essential oils** – Peppermint and lavender are some of the best essential oils that you can add to your body butter recipe. Aside from making your skin look more radiant and fresh, these ingredients can also soothe your scalp, reduce dandruff, and prevent irritations from occurring.

## Myth 4: Body butter is not safe for pregnancy

This statement is false. In fact, body butter is highly recommended for use by pregnant women. This natural cosmetic product can help reduce the stretch marks and maintain the skin's softness while your belly starts to expand. A combination of shea butter, Vitamin E, and lavender oil will ensure that your belly will be properly moisturized while it is stretching.

However, you need to make sure that the body butter that you will use is devoid of any ingredients that might cause any allergic reaction to your body.

For best results, you should apply this natural product thrice a day. This will ensure that your skin will maintain its smoothness. If you consistently use body butter for pregnancy, your skin cells will stay supple, yet firm.

## Myth 5: You need to apply large amounts of body butter in order to gain the best results.

Not necessarily. Even if you have scaly and extremely dry skin, you only need a few spoonfuls of body butter every day. The important thing to remember is to apply it constantly. For people who already have a smooth skin, you can apply body butter once or twice a day in order to maintain its good condition. But for those who are experiencing severe dryness, you need to apply body butter three to four times a day to ensure quicker results.

## Myth 6: You do not need to add preservatives on beauty products

Body butter contains water and several nutrients. This makes it a good breeding ground for bacteria and fungi. If you do not properly preserve your product, it will become spoiled and unusable. If you accidentally use these products, it might cause skin infections.

If you are feeling uncomfortable with adding chemical preservatives in your body butter recipe, there are a lot of natural ingredients that you can use as alternatives. They are as effective as their chemical counterparts, and they are safe for people with sensitive skin.

## Myth 7: I can't use body butter on my kids

The good news is natural body butters are safe for your children. Shea body butter, for instance, can be applied to your babies in order to protect their very delicate skin. It is recommended if you use it on their bottoms so that they will not experience diaper rash. This product can also be used to massage their bodies. And if they have eczema, you can apply body butter on the affected parts so that these will heal quickly. Just make sure that the body butter does not contain any ingredients that might cause any allergic reaction to their bodies.

# Conclusion

Thank you again for purchasing this book!

I hope this book was able to help you to start having great skin with very little efforts and cost by making your all-natural, easy to make body butters.

The next step is to enjoy that flawless and smooth skin. Share the secret to others too, by sharing this book to them.

Finally, if you enjoyed this book, please take the time to share your thoughts and post a review on Amazon. We do our best to reach out to readers and provide the best value we can. Your positive review will help us achieve that. It'd be greatly appreciated!

Thank you and good luck!

# Check Out My Other Books

Below you'll find some of my other popular books that are popular on Amazon and Kindle as well. Simply click on the links below to check them out. Alternatively, you can visit my author page on Amazon to see other work done by me.

Coconut Oil for Easy Weight Loss: A Step by Step Guide for Using Virgin Coconut Oil for Quick and Easy Weight Loss

http://www.amazon.com/Coconut-Oil-Easy-Weight-Loss-ebook/dp/B00JG8H8DE

Superfoods that Kickstart Your Weight Loss Learn How to Use 30 Superfoods to Boost Weight Loss, Immunity and to Live a Healthier Lifestyle

http://www.amazon.com/Superfoods-that-Kickstart-Your-Weight-ebook/dp/B00JNAPM9M

Carrier Oils for Beginners: Discover the Characteristics and Beauty and Health Benefits of Carrier Oils For mixing Aromatherapy Essential Oils

http://www.amazon.com/Carrier-Oils-Beginners-Characteristics-Aromatherapy-ebook/dp/B00K88GI2S

Natural Homemade Cleaning Recipes For Beginners: Essential Oil Recipes For Household Cleaning, Laundry & Toxic Free Living http://www.amazon.com/Natural-Homemade-Cleaning-Recipes-Beginners-ebook/dp/B00K87UBQI

The Best Secrets of Natural Remedies: The Ultimate Guide to Natural Remedies to Prevent and Cure Illnesses, Cold and Flu for Your Family

http://www.amazon.com/Best-Secrets-Natural-Remedies-Illnesses-ebook/dp/B00JNDCOCM

The Hypothyroidism Handbook:An Everyday Guide to Natural Solutions of living with Hypothyroidism including increased energy, lasting weight loss, and general well-being

http://www.amazon.com/Hypothyroidism-Handbook-Solutions- including-increased-ebook/dp/B00JNIGIV0

The Hyperthyroidism Handbook: An Everyday Guide to Natural Solutions of Living with Hyperthyroidism including Weight Gain, Increased Energy and General Well-being

http://www.amazon.com/Hyperthyroidism-Handbook-Solutions-including-Hypothyroidism-ebook/dp/B00JOHU5SM

Essential Oils & Weight Loss for Beginners: Ultimate Guide to Losing Weight, Increasing Energy, Balancing Metabolism & Appetite Using Essential Oils & Aromatherapy

http://www.amazon.com/Essential-Oils-Weight-Loss-Beginners-ebook/dp/B00JOFOWP6

Top Essential Oil Recipes: A Recipe Guide Of Natural, Non-Toxic Aromatherapy & Essential Oils for Healing Common Ailments, Beauty, Stress & Anxiety

http://www.amazon.com/Top-Essential-Oil-Recipes-Aromatherapy-ebook/dp/B00JY434E2

Soap Making For Beginners: A Guide to Making Natural Homemade Soaps from Scratch, Includes Recipes and Step by Step Processes for Making Soaps

http://www.amazon.com/Soap-Making-Beginners-Homemade-Processes-ebook/dp/B00JYKH75I

Body Butters For Beginners: Proven Secrets To Making All Natural Body Butters For Rejuvenating And Hydrating Your Skin

http://www.amazon.com/Body-Butters-Beginners-Rejuvenating-Hydrating-ebook/dp/B00K6LVV6A

Apple Cider Vinegar For Beginners: Proven Secrets Using Apple Cider Vinegar For Health, Weight Loss, and Skin Care

http://www.amazon.com/Apple-Cider-Vinegar-Beginners-Aromatherapy-ebook/dp/B00K6YY6HI

Homemade Body Scrubs & Masks For Beginners: 50 Proven All Natural, Easy Recipes For Body & Facial Masks To Exfoliate Nourish, & Care For Your Skin

http://www.amazon.com/Homemade-Body-Scrubs-Masks-Beginners-ebook/dp/B00K79D4SY

Essential Oils Box Set #1: Essential Oils & Weight Loss For Beginners (Ultimate Guide to Losing Weight, Increasing Energy, Balancing Metabolism & Appetite Using Essential Oils & Aromatherapy) + Top Essential Oil Recipes (A Recipe Guide of Natural, Non-Toxic Aromatherapy & Essential Oils for Healing Common Ailments, Beauty, Stress & Anxiety)

http://www.amazon.com/ESSENTIAL-OILS-BOX-SET-Aromatherapy-ebook/dp/B00K7Q8HRK

Essential Oils Box Set #2: Essential Oils & Weight Loss For Beginners (Ultimate Guide to Losing Weight, Increasing Energy, Balancing Metabolism & Appetite Using Essential Oils & Aromatherapy) + Top Essential Oil Recipes (A Recipe Guide of Natural, Non-Toxic Aromatherapy & Essential Oils for Healing Common Ailments, Beauty, Stress & Anxiety)

http://www.amazon.com/ESSENTIAL-OILS-BOX-SET-Aromatherapy-ebook/dp/B00K7Q8HRK

Box Set#3: Coconut Oil for Easy Weight Loss(A Step by Step Guide for Using Virgin Coconut Oil for Quick and Easy Weight Loss) + Apple Cider Vinegar(Proven Secrets Using Apple Cider Vinegar for Health, Weight Loss, and Skin Care)

http://www.amazon.com/Box-Set-Beginners-Aromatherapy-Essential-ebook/dp/B00K9TEGUW

Box Set #4: Body butters For Beginners(Proven Secrets To Making All Natural Body Butters For Rejuvenating And Hydrating Your Skin) & Top Essential Oil Recipes: A Recipe Guide Of Natural, Non-Toxic Aromatherapy & Essential Oils for Healing Common Ailments, Beauty, Stress & Anxiety

http://www.amazon.com/Box-Set-Butters-Beginners-Essential-ebook/dp/B00KA02F4Y

Box Set #5: Soap Making For Beginners(A Guide to Making Natural Homemade Soaps from Scratch, Includes Recipes and Step by Step Processes for Making Soaps) + Homemade Body Scrubs & Masks For Beginners(50 Proven All Natural, Easy Recipes For Body Scrub & Facial Masks To Efoliate, Nourish, & Care For Your Skin)

http://www.amazon.com/Box-Set-Beginners-Homemade-Recipes-ebook/dp/B00K9U3I2I

Box Set #6: Body Butters for Beginners (Proven Secrets To Making All Natural Body Butters For Rejuvenating And Hydrating Your Skin) +Homemade Body Scrubs & Masks For Beginners(50 Proven All Natural, Easy Recipes For Body Scrub & Facial Masks To Exfoliate, Nourish, & Care For Your Skin)

http://www.amazon.com/Box-Set-Beginners-Exfoliating-Moisturizing-ebook/dp/B00K9U3Y4O

Box Set #7: TOP ESSENTIAL OILS(A Recipe Guide Of Natural, Non-Toxic Aromatherapy & Essential Oils For Healing, Common Ailments, Beauty, Stress & Anxiety) & THE BEST SECRETS OF NATURAL REMEDIES(The Ultimate Guide to Natural Remedies to Prevent and Cure Illnesses, Cold and Flu for Your Family)

http://www.amazon.com/BOX-SET-Essential-Recipes-Remedies-ebook/dp/B00K9WPMQG

Box Set #8: NATURAL HOMEMADE CLEANING RECIPES FOR BEGINNERS (Essential Oil Recipes for Household Cleaning, Laundry & Toxic Free Living) + TOP ESSENTIAL OILS(A Recipe Guide Of Natural, Non-Toxic Aromatherapy

& Essential Oils For Healing, Common Ailments, Beauty, Stress & Anxiety)

http://www.amazon.com/BOX-SET-Beginners-Essential-Aromatherapy-ebook/dp/B00KAMNGBS

Box Set #9: Essential Oils & Weight Loss for Beginners (Ultimate Guide to Losing Weight, Increasing Energy, Balancing Metabolism & Appetite Using Essential Oils & Aromatherapy) + Carrier Oils for Beginners (Discover the Characteristics and Beauty and Health Benefits of Carrier Oils for Mixing Aromatherapy Essential Oils)

http://www.amazon.com/BOX-SET-Essential-Beginners-Aromatherapy-ebook/dp/B00KAODL6Q

BOX SET #10: THE HYPERTHYROIDISM HANDBOOK (An Everyday Guide to Natural Solutions of Living with Hyperthyroidism including Weight Gain, Increased Energy and General Well-being) + THE HYPOTHYROIDISM HANDBOOK (Everyday Guide to Natural Solutions of Living With Hypothyroidism Including Increased Energy, Lasting Weight Loss, and General Well-Being)

http://www.amazon.com/BOX-SET-10-Hyperthyroidism-Hypothyroidism-ebook/dp/B00KAKMSBY

BOX SET #11: CARRIER OILS FOR BEGINNERS (Discover the Characteristics and Beauty and Health Benefits of Carrier Oils for Mixing Aromatherapy Essential Oils) + Essential Oils & Aromatherapy for Beginners (Secrets to Beauty, Health and Weight Loss Using Proven Essential Oil and Aromatherapy Recipes http://www.amazon.com/BOX-SET-Beginners-Essential-Aromatherapy-ebook/dp/B00KAONEQ8

BOX SET 12: ESSENTIAL OILS & WEIGHT LOSS FOR BEGINNERS: (Ultimate Guide to Losing Weight, Increasing Energy, Balancing Metabolism & Appetite Using Essential Oils & Aromatherapy) + TOP ESSENTIAL OIL RECIPES (A Recipe Guide of Natural, Non-Toxic Aromatherapy & Essential Oils for Healing Common Ailments, Beauty, Stress & Anxiety) + CARRIER OILS FOR BEGINNERS (Discover the Characteristics & Beauty & Health Benefits of Carrier Oils for Mixing Aromatherapy Essential Oils) + ESSENTIAL OILS & AROMATHERAPY FOR BEGINNERS (Secrets to Beauty & weight Loss Using Proven Essential Oil & Aromatherapy Recipes) + NATURAL HOMEMADE CLEANING RECIPES FOR BEGINNERS (Essential Oil Recipes for Household Cleaning, Laundry & Toxic Free Living)

http://www.amazon.com/BOX-SET-12-Essential-Aromatherapy-ebook/dp/B00KCBCHE4

BOX SET #13: SUPERFOODS THAT KICKSTART YOUR WEIGHT LOSS (Learn How to Use 30 Superfoods to Boost Weight Loss, Immunity and to Live a Healthier Lifestyle) + ESSENTIAL OILS & AROMATHERAPY FOR BEGINNERS (Secrets to Beauty, Health and Weight Loss Using Proven Essential Oil and Aromatherapy Recipes) + BODY BUTTERS FOR BEGINNERS (Proven Secrets To Making All Natural Body Butters For Rejuvenating And Hydrating Your Skin) + SOAP MAKING FOR BEGINNERS (A Guide to Making Natural Homemade Soaps from Scratch, Includes Recipes and Step by Step Processes for Making Soaps) +

HOMEMADE BODY SCRUBS FOR BEGINNERS (50 Proven All Natural, Easy Recipes For Body Scrub & Facial Masks To Exfoliate, Nourish, & Care For Your Skin)

http://www.amazon.com/BOX-SET-Superfoods-Kickstart-Aromatherapy-ebook/dp/B00KC8G6DK/


BOX SET 14: Essential Oils & Weight Loss for Beginners (Ultimate Guide to Losing Weight, Increasing Energy, Balancing Metabolism & Appetite Using Essential Oils & Aromatherapy) + Apple Cider Vinegar for Beginners (Proven Secrets Using Apple Cider Vinegar for Health, Weight Loss, and Skin Care) + Body Butters For Beginners (Proven Secrets To Making All Natural Body Butters For Rejuvenating And Hydrating Your Skin)
+ Homemade Body Scrubs & Masks for Beginners (50 Proven All Natural, Easy Recipes for Body Scrub & Facial Masks to Exfoliate, Nourish, & Care for Your Skin) + Coconut Oil for Easy Weight Loss (A Step by Step Guide for Using Virgin Coconut Oil for Quick and Easy Weight Loss)

http://www.amazon.com/BOX-SET-Essential-Beginners-Aromatherapy-ebook/dp/B00KEDO68U

www.ingramcontent.com/pod-product-compliance
Lightning Source LLC
Chambersburg PA
CBHW060219290526
45789CB00003B/1332